Intermittent Fasting

Lose Fat, Build Muscle, and Get Fit

Table of Contents

Introduction

Congratulations on downloading your copy of *Intermittent Fasting: Lose Fat, Build Muscle, and Get Fit*. Thank you for doing so.

Intermittent fasting has grown in popularity in recent years, thanks in large part to its ability to promote greater rates of nutrient absorption in the meals you eat. It has also grown in popularity because it doesn't require adherents to change radically the types of foods you are eating, when you are eating, or even drastically alter the number of calories you consume in each 24-hour period. In fact, the most common type of intermittent fasting is to simply consume two slightly larger than average meals during a day instead of the usual three.

This makes the intermittent fasting diet plan an ideal choice for those who find they have difficulty sticking to more stringent diet plans, as it only requires changing one habit, the number of meals per day, instead of many habits all at once. Many people find that practicing intermittent fasting leads to real results. It's simple enough to manage successfully over a prolonged period while at the same time being efficient enough to provide the type of results that can keep motivation levels high enough once the novelty of the new diet begins to fade.

The secret to intermittent fasting's success is the simple fact that your body behaves differently when it's in a fasting, versus a fed state. When your body is in what is known as a fed state, it is actively digesting and absorbing food. This begins some five minutes after you have finished putting food into your body, and can last anywhere from three to five hours depending on the how complicated the food is for your body to digest. While in the fed state, your body is actively producing insulin which in turn makes it harder for it to burn fat properly.

The period after digestion has occurred, the insulin levels start dropping back towards normal which can take anywhere from 8 to 12 hours, and is the buffer between the fed and fasted state. Once your insulin levels return to normal, the fasted state begins which is the period where your body can process fat most effectively. Unfortunately, this means that many people never reach the point where they can burn fat most efficiently, as they rarely go eight hours, much less 12 hours from some type of caloric consumption. There is hope! However, as to start seeing real results, all you need to do is break the three meal a day habit.

There are plenty of books on this subject on the market. Thanks again for choosing this one. Every effort was made to ensure it is full of as much useful information as possible. Please enjoy!

Chapter 1: How Intermittent Fasting Works

History of Intermittent Fasting

Fasting is not a trend and has been a part of some religious beliefs including Buddhism, Islam, and Christianity. Decades before this generation, the process may have been because of the unavailability of food resources. Just remember, it is not a starvation diet since starvation is considered an involuntary absence of food. Consider breakfast which is the most important time of your day. After all, it is 'break-fast'—which is a part of every day.

Fasting dates to the day of Hippocrates of Cos {c460 – c370BC} who is considered in many ideals as the father of modern medicine. He stated, "To eat when you are sick is to feed your illness." Plato, an ancient Greek thinker, and Aristotle, his student, were believers and supporters of fasting. The Greeks believed that fasting is the "physician within." This is the same logic/instinct portrayed by your pets.

Ben Franklin, an important founding father of America, also stated, "The best of all medicine is resting and fasting."

The Basics

Intermittent fasting is a way of eating to ensure that you get the most out of every meal you eat. The core tenants of intermittent fasting mean that you don't need to change what you are eating. Instead, you must change when you are eating it. Intermittent fasting is a viable alternative to traditional diets or simply cutting your daily caloric intake which can help fasters lean up without changing the number of calories they consume in a day. In fact, the preferred method of intermittent fasting is to simply eat two large meals every day instead of three (or more) meals in that same period.

Intermittent fasting is also a great option for those who traditionally have trouble sticking to diet plans since it only requires you to change one small habit, instead of several larger ones. Intermittent fasting is extremely effective for most people because it is simple enough for them to attempt. At the same time, it is efficient to warrant the task.

The key to understating why intermittent fasting is so successful lies in the differences in your body during a fasted state versus a fed state, as well as the important changes that will come across because of changing habits and sticking with it.

The body is considered to be in the fed state when it is in the process of absorbing and digesting food. The fed state tends to start roughly five minutes after you begin eating, and lasting from three to five hours, depending on how long it takes your body to digest the meal. A fed state, in turn, leads to higher levels of insulin which make it much more difficult for the body to burn fat. The period directly after the fed sate is referred to as the post-absorptive state which is the period of time where the body is not actively processing food, and its insulin levels begin to fall. This state lasts for between eight and twelve hours and directly precedes the fasted state.

The fasted state occurs between nine and twelve hours after the post-absorptive state and is the point where the body's insulin levels are at its lowest which in turn make it the period of time where the most fat can be burned during physical activity. Unfortunately for many people, they rarely go twelve hours without eating which means that no matter how hard they exercise they are not burning fat as efficiently as possible. However, this also means that you can burn fat and build muscle by simply altering your feeding habits.

Scientifically Proven

Your metabolic rate is increased with short-term fasting because of the hormonal changes ranging in categories of 3.6% to 14%. Studies have established weight loss after three to twenty-four weeks on the intermittent fasting program to maintain losses of 3.0 to 8.0%. In comparison to other studies on weight loss, these are high percentages that cannot be ignored.

In the same studies, many of the individuals lost 4.0 to 7.0% of his/her waist circumference. This is an indication of how the harmful buildup of belly fat can cause disease and other issues around your organs. You have to consider these results are from eating fewer overall calories, and not binging during the days off. You must maintain a sensible eating program.

While the science behind intermittent fasting is certainly promising, there are a few things you will need to keep in mind when starting any new dietary plan. No diet, regardless of how miraculous it appears, can help you if you don't obey a few golden rules.

- *Keep a calorie deficit:* While this is true for any diet, it is even more true for intermittent fasting since it can be so easy to overeat once you do eat in such a way that it negates any benefits you might have felt. Remember, you need to burn 3,500 calories weekly to lose one pound each week.

- *Maintain self-control:* Intermittent fasting only works if your body goes completely without food for at least twelve hours, any caloric intact resets the cycle. As such, it is extremely important to ensure that you maintain control of you bodily urges if you hope to see real results from this type of approach. Remember, fasting for at least twelve hours only allows you to eat normally or slightly more than an average meal, it does not give you license to eat everything in sight. Keeping your appetites in check is a strict requirement for success.

- *Be consistent:* Regardless of the type of weight loss that you ultimately choose to pursue, it is important to choose one and stick with it. Attempting an intermittent fast for a few days before switching to another plan such as the Paleo diet before trying out a low-carb approach will only cause your body to freak out and hold on to every possible calorie until it figures out what in the world is happening.

Remember, fasting regularly and consistently is the surest way to see any of its benefits. Only after your body has time to adjust to your new routine will it then be able to adapt appropriately. It can begin to increase several positive enzymes and neural pathways to maximize weight loss using this method. Consider consistency the ace-in-the-hole of proactive weight loss success.

Possible Side Effects:

While intermittent fasting has some scientifically proven benefits, it is not with its potential side effects. The biggest one of these is the initial change in your bowel movements as periods of constipation or in some cases diarrhea could occur. Fortunately, they should not last more than a few days as your body adjusts to the new method of caloric intake.

Additional damage can be done to the body if periods of fasting are routinely followed by periods of excessive binging. It is important to attempt intermittent fasting, and your periods of eating after, in moderation. If you notice any serious immediate physical changes after you begin any form of dieting regime, it is important to consult a nutritionist.

Chapter 2: Intermittent Types and Fasting Schedules

While the core ideas behind the various forms of intermittent fasting are all the same, there are quite a few different ways to go about it. Your best bet is to try a few and see which one your body naturally responds to the easiest.

16:8 Method

This method involves fasting for 16 hours for men, or 14 hours for women, before allowing a reasonable number of calories for the remaining 8 to 10 hours. During this period, you should only consume items that have zero calories including black coffee (a splash of cream is fine), water, diet soda, and sugar-free gum. The easiest way to attempt this schedule is to stop eating after dinner in the evening and wait 14 or 16 hours from there. This means skipping breakfast and picking things up in the early afternoon.

Again, the specifics of when you fast are not nearly as important as ensuring that you fast for the same period of time as regularly as possible. If you vary your fasting period too much, it can lead to an erratic change in your hormones, which among other things; make it much more difficult for your body to shed any excess weight. If you find yourself without the time required to eat a proper meal to break the fast normally, ensure you at least eat something to keep your body on the correct cycle.

If you are exercising, as well as intermittently fasting, it is important to ensure that you are eating more carbohydrates than fats while you are working out, while on days you are not exercising the opposite is true. It is important to ensure that every day you keep your protein intake at a steady level. Stay away from processed foods whenever possible.

One of the biggest benefits of this type of fasting is that it's extremely flexible so that it will work for a wide variety schedules. Most people find it helpful to either eat two large meals during the 8 or 10-hour period feeding period or split that time into three smaller meals as that is the way most people are already programmed.

On days you are exercising as well as fasting, it is important to try and always break your fast with a mix of protein, vegetables, and fruit. If you generally go to the gym directly after you have broken your fast, it is important to include enough carbohydrates to give your muscles the energy they need to get the most out of your workout.

If you are planning to exercise, it is usually best to start the early afternoon healthy with a medium calorie meal. Then, exercise within three hours before eating a larger meal soon afterward. In this larger meal, it is important to add a larger portion of complex carbohydrates. You can even have a little dessert as long as it is in moderation. Remember, fasting is different than dieting.

On days you do not plan on exercising, it is important to adjust your caloric intake appropriately. Start by limiting your carbohydrate intake, and instead focus on eating lots of protein, dark green, leafy vegetables and fruit in moderation. Unlike on days you are exercising, the first meal you eat on rest days should be your largest regarding caloric intake with this one meal counting for about 40 percent of your daily total.

Remember, during this meal, you should be taking in more protein than anything else. For your final meal during rest days, it is important to include a protein source that will take lots of time to digest which in turn means it will keep you full for more of your fast the following morning. It also provides the body with enough stored amino acids to prevent it from breaking down muscle during the fast.

Eat-Stop-Eat

This form of fasting can be considered the most beneficial to those who are already eating healthy but want to give their weight loss an extra boost. On this type of program, you don't eat anything one or two days a week. During this period, you should only consume things that have zero calories including black coffee (a splash of cream is fine), water, diet soda, and sugar-free gum.

When you are finished fasting, it is important not to eat too much more than normal and always to avoid binging as extended periods of fast/binge cycles can cause serious damage to your body. As always, it is important to practice moderation and self-control to get the most out of the fasting cycle.

This fast cycle works on the assumption that in to lose a pound of weight a week, all you need to do is give up 3,500 calories. So, it might be best to get it out of the way in two quick bursts rather than fasting for a portion of every single day. This fasting plan emphasizes resistance weight training for maximum benefits.

Going a full day without eating can be difficult for some people at first, but it is perfectly acceptable to work up to a full day of fasting by holding out as long as possible and increasing that amount of time with practice. A good way to start is by choosing days that you know don't have any prior food commitments. Beginning a fasting program on a day when you know you have a lunch meeting is just a bad idea.

When first starting this fast cycle, fatigue, headaches or feelings of anger or anxiousness are all common side-effects and should be considered a good stopping point for your current fast. These side-effects will diminish as your body adjusts to the new cycle.

After going a full day without any calories, it will be natural to have the desire to binge during your fist meal. You must have the self-control to fight these urges since not only is binging bad for you; it can easily undo all your hard work from the previous 24 hours. Practice self-discipline and make your fasting worth the effort.

The Warrior Diet

The Warrior Diet takes the 16:8 Program and kicks it up a notch by recommending that you fast for roughly 20 hours out of each day followed by one meal where you get all your calories in the four remaining hours of the day.

This form of intermittent fasting follows the belief that humans are naturally nocturnal eaters. Therefore, eating at night helps the body more easily process the nutrients it needs. In this case, fasting is a bit of a misnomer as during the 20-hour period you are allowed to eat a serving of raw vegetables or fruits and maybe a serving of protein if you just can't otherwise continue.

This works because it causes the body's natural sympathetic nervous system to activate a flight or fight response which in turns increases your natural levels of alertness, and increases energy while at the same time increasing the amount of fat burned. The large meal each evening then allows the body to focus on repairing itself and improving its muscles. When following the Warrior Diet, it is important to start each evening meal with vegetables, followed by protein, fat, and carbohydrates.

This form of fasting is popular for two reasons. First, the fact that a few small and reasonable snacks are allowed during the fasting process making this type of fasting attractive to those who are attempting the practice for the first time. Second, nearly everyone who attempts this form of fasting reports a significant amount of increased energy throughout the day as well as increase in the amount of fat lost per week.

On the other hand, the relatively strict nature of this diet can make it difficult for some people to follow for long periods of time. The timing of the large meal can also make it difficult for some people to follow because it can naturally interfere with some social engagements. Finally, some people don't like having to eat their food in a specific order. Try it for yourself and see what works for you.

Fat Loss Forever

This form of intermittent fasting combines elements of several other styles of fasting to create something rather unique. The good news is that you get a cheat day every week. The bad news is that it is followed by a one and a half day fast with the remainder of the week being split between 16:8 and 20:4 fasting.

For this diet, it is important to schedule your exercise rest days for the second part of the 36-hour cycle. Otherwise, it is important to stay as busy on these days as possible to help combat your hunger. If you find it hard to control your appetite on cheat days, then this form of intermittent fasting may not be for you since it requires you to go from sixty to zero quickly and regularly.

Also, it is important not to try and last 36 hours without eating food all at once. You will need to build up your body's tolerance for fasting. As such, it is usually better to start with another form of intermittent fasting and work up to the Fat Loss Forever method after your body has already gotten out of the habit of eating every three or four hours.

Remember to always fast responsibly, and never push your body to the point where you feel physically ill. Also, remember it is important to fast on a routine to allow your body the time it needs to adjust to the change.

Alternate Day Diet

This form of intermittent fasting actually means you never have to go long without food, if you so choose. Every other day you eat normally, and on the off-days, you simply consume one-fifth of the calories you consume on the normal days. The average daily caloric consumption is between 2,000 and 2,500 calories which mean that the average off-day varies between 400 and 500 calories. If you enjoy exercising every day, then this form of intermittent fasting may not be for you since you will have to severely limit your workouts on off-days.

When you first start this form of intermittent fasting, the easiest way to make it through the low-calorie days is by trying any one of a variety of protein shakes. It is important to work back to 'real' natural foods on these days because they will always be healthier than the shakes.

This form of intermittent fasting is all about losing weight. Those who try it tend to average between two and three pounds lost per week. If you attempt the Alternate Day Diet, it is extremely important to eat regularly on your full-calorie days. Binging will not only negate any progress you have made, but it can also cause serious damage to your body if continued over time.

Irregularly Skipping Meals

If you are interested in trying out the benefits of intermittent fasting for yourself, but you have an irregular schedule or are not sure if it is for you, then skipping a meal or two now and then may be the type of intermittent fasting for you. As previously discussed, getting into a fasting routine is important to see the maximum results for your effort, but that doesn't mean occasionally fasting doesn't come with some benefits as well.

What's more, once you have tried skipping a meal now and then you can see for yourself just how easy it is which in turn can lead to more positive changes down the line. With so many intermittent fasting options available the odds are good that one fits your schedule, so give it a try. What have you got to lose (besides a few pounds)?

Chapter 3: Health Benefits

Other than weight loss, you can receive benefits from intermittent fasting in many other ways. You will live a longer life from achieving an extended fasting state and diverting your energy while improving your biological functions.

Just remember, the plan will not in any way cause you to starve. The emergency signals transported by your body is simply that— a signal. The fasting state your body is experiencing will diminish once your body adjusts to the diet method of intermittent fasting you choose to take.

These are some of the crucial elements to consider:

- *Brain Health:* Your brain hormone—BDNF—also known as brain-derived "neurotropic" factor—is a protein that can aid in the growth of new nerve cells. It is also believed to provide protection against Alzheimer's and Parkinson's disease.

- *Cancer:* Studies using animals have suggested intermittent fasting can be beneficial in the prevention of cancer.

- *Heart Health:* The blood triglycerides, LDL cholesterol, insulin resistance, and blood sugar can be reduced using this plan. Each of these presents a huge risk element for heart ailments or disease.

- *Inflammation:* Chronic diseases are driven by inflammation, and the fasting plans help to reduce the inflammation as proven by private studies. Your body will be capable of repairing, healing, and recovering more quickly than without the diet plan.

- *Insulin Resistance:* Your blood sugar levels can be lowered by 3.0% to 3.6 as fasting insulin levels can also decrease as much as 20% to 31%. These figures indicate you should be better sheltered against type 2 diabetes as well as a more continuous level of mood and energy stages.

- *Anti-Aging:* The process has only been tested using animals, but the rats tested lived 36% to 83% longer than ones that were not fasting.

- *Lower Stress Levels:* The cortisol production is lowered.

- *Fatty Acid Oxidation:* Your body will burn more fats as energy with the oxidation process and will also provide quick weight loss.

Note: Each of these studies are in early stages. More research needs to be provided using human testing during the fasting process.

Chapter 4: The Process

While intermittent fasting is undeniably beneficial, it can be difficult to get started or to see through to the point where your body adapts to a new schedule. The following tips and tricks can help set you on the path to success.

Have a conversation with yourself:
Intermittent fasting has a wide variety of proven benefits, but it is not for everyone. Before you attempt a fast, it is important to have a real dialogue with yourself. Consider your level of self-discipline, your current attachment to food, any regular activities that would make fasting difficult or awkward, your general lifestyle, and your level of exercise. Deciding to try a different fitness regime is a lot easier on day one, than after struggling through a week or more of faulty fasting.

Watch your response:
While it is important to keep tabs on how your body is responding to intermittent fasting, it is doubly important to monitor your vitals during the initial phase when your body is adjusting to the new feeding times. Some discomfort is to be expected for the first three to four weeks, but anything longer or more severe should be discussed with a doctor as soon as possible.

The early days will have ups and downs:
While your body adjusts to intermittent fasting, there will be times where you are losing weight and times where your body is trying to hold on to every calorie it has. This is natural and to be expected as your body realigns its hormone levels.

Drink lots of water:
Not only will water help you feel full throughout your fast, staying hydrated is akin to staying healthy. Aim for at least a gallon of water per day.

Caffeine naturally suppresses the appetite:
Black coffee works best as there is little to it which can negatively affect your metabolism or general wellbeing. The same cannot be said for most 0-calorie caffeinated beverages.

Artificial sweeteners have been shown to cause some health problems. Still, anything with caffeine will help calm your appetite for at least a little while.

Keep yourself busy:
Ensure that the latter parts of your fast aren't just spent waiting around to eat. Intermittent fasting has the possibility to be either extremely difficult or surprisingly easy depending solely on how much of the time you spend thinking about food. Find ways to occupy your mind, and you will be surprised how quickly meal time will roll around.

Start each fast off right:
At the start of your fast, your body will still have the most fuel in its system to work with, which is why it is best to start each fast with the most difficult items on your to-do list. As you move farther and farther from the last period of time, and you take in fresh calories, your thought processes will naturally begin to slow in your body's effort to save energy. Difficult tasks will inherently seem easier when your body is working at maximum efficiency.

Make it work for you:
Intermittent fasting can work around any type of schedule which is part of what makes it so great. If you find yourself feeling trapped by the period of time you are allowing yourself to eat, why don't you move it? Fasting should be about adding freedom to your schedule, not restraining it.

Don't expect results overnight:
As previously discussed, it will take some time for your body to adjust fully to your new dietary patterns, and for it to start reflecting these new results. Try intermittent fasting regularly for at least a month before rendering judgment on the success of the plan.

Vary your schedule:
After you have given your body time to adjust to an intermittent fasting schedule, it is important to take the time to fluctuate your on/off patterns throughout the day to see what works best

for you. Taking the time to experiment may yield unexpected results.

Start slow:
If you find that you are having difficulty starting the transition to an intermittent fasting program full bore, try moving your breakfast time back one hour each week. Before you know it, you will have reached a 16:8 or 14:10 split without even trying.

Keep it to yourself:
While there is plenty of scientific evidence that supports intermittent fasting, there are still plenty of skeptics out there. That negativity isn't something you need, especially when you are first starting out. After you have started seeing results for yourself, it will be much easier to defend the process to non-believers. Just show them a before and after picture.

Start the day off with a belly full of liquid:
Often the signals for hunger and the signals for thirst can get crossed in your brain. After it has sent out enough ignored thirst signals, it starts sending out hunger signals instead. As such, starting the morning off by drinking at least half a liter of water is an excellent way to quench your body's thirst from the past seven or eight hours. It should be enough to keep you feeling full for at least a few extra hours each morning.

Don't take on too much, too fast: Even if you think you feel fine when you first begin an intermittent fast cycle, it is important to always give your body the time it needs to recover. Never go more than two days out of a week without eating. There is an important distinction between fasting and starving yourself.

Splurge when you want:
Remember that you need to burn 3,500 calories to lose a pound a week, but how you do that is up to you. If you want to have a particularly appetizing dessert or unhealthy main course, that is perfectly fine, as long as you make an effort to make up the difference throughout the week.

Distract yourself:
Distraction is especially important as your body is adapting to your new eating habits, and becomes increasingly important the farther into a fast you go. Try going out and being active when you are struggling with the plan to help refocus your thinking patterns. Besides, the exercise also helps push away the pounds.

Add protein to your meals:
There is nothing better at combating hunger than protein, plain and simple. It is also great for building lean muscle. If you find yourself unable to get through even 10 hours without eating, then it might be a sign that you should add more protein to your diet.

Try Branched Chain Amino Acids:
For those on a low-calorie diet such as intermittent fasting, studies show that a BCAA supplement will stimulate additional fat loss while at the same time preventing lean muscle from being consumed as the body tries to feed itself.

Intermittent fasting is not an excuse to eat poorly:
Intermittent fasting works on the principle that eating fewer calories than you burn is a surefire way to lose weight. This theory falls apart if you use the fact that you are fasting as an excuse to eat nothing but junk food when you are eating. Self-control and self-discipline are both equally important when it comes to eating properly. Intermittent fasting has a wide variety of health benefits. Why not accentuate them even more with a healthy diet to go along with it?

Break your fast the right way:
The content and quality of your first meal of the day can easily set the tone for those that follow. Use this to your advantage, and start your feeding window off right with something fit and healthy. You will be surprised at how much this improves your willpower for later meals.

Consider the difference between head hunger and body hunger:
As you get used to the process of intermittent fasting, you will become acquainted with several different types of hunger and ultimately learn how to tell when you are truly hungry as

opposed to just habitually used to eating. While it will initially be difficult to tell the difference, you will come to know them both intimately in time.

Learn what your body is saying: While many people consider a sudden craving for a particular type of food as an indication that they are hungry, and take action to respond accordingly. This, in fact, is often just a craving brought on by an ancient part of the brain which equates things that are salty, sweet, and high in fat as vital parts of a regular diet. Since once upon a time, having those three qualities equated to things that were high in positive nutrients as well. This is no longer the case and tends to be the opposite these days. As such, these types of urges can safely be ignored. Take the time to investigate a sudden surge of hunger to see if it could instead be related to your emotional state instead of your physical one.

Exercise in moderation:
Dieting works by ensuring that you are taking in fewer calories than you are burning in a fixed period of time. As such, if you are trying one of the intermittent fasting options that involve you not eating for a day or more, then it is extremely important to ensure that you adjust your exercise plan for these days as well. When exercising, your body requires fuel. It will take it from your muscles if you don't give it another choice. Exercising too much while you're fasting is a guaranteed recipe for disaster.

Don't cover real issues with fasting:
Those with a penchant for eating disorders or those who believe they might be should stay away for intermittent fasting as it can easily lead to more serious issues if not controlled properly. Remember, it is important to have the willpower to stop eating for a set period of time, but it is also equally important to have the willpower to begin eating again once the fast is over.

Chapter 5: Weight Loss and Intermittent Fasting

You need to understand what your daily calorie needs will be to adopt a realistic diet plan and maintain a new desirable weight. The use of an adult <u>BMI and Calorie Calculator</u> will be an essential tool if the calories are not indicated in the recipe. Most products you purchase will have ingredient panels listing the counts, so you will have a general idea of how to plan your menu around your intermittent fasting plan.

You will need to enter your sex, height, weight, and age into the calculator. You will also need to provide the calculator with your daily activity schedule (such as daily—more than an hour—less than an hour—or rarely. The BMI will indicate your BMI score and the amount of calories necessary to maintain your current body weight. It will make your goals simpler to map by providing you with the tallies from your calculations to lower your counts.

Maintain a Healthy Diet Plan

The components for a healthier eating pattern using intermittent fasting methods will account for all the beverages and foods within a suitable calorie level. A good plan for a healthy fasting pattern will include the following:

- Whole Fruits

- Oils

- Grains (a minimum of half should be whole grains)

- Protein foods such as eggs, poultry, lean meats, seafood, nuts, seeds, and soy products

- Varied veggies from all the main subgroups include— starchy legumes (peas and beans), red and orange, dark green and others.

Health concerns in the United States are focused on fundamental elements that should be limited when using the intermittent fasting diet plan. They recommend you do the following:

- Consume less than 10% of your daily calories from saturated fats.

- Eat less than 10% of your daily intake of calories from added sugars.

- Sodium consumption should be less than 2,300 mg (milligrams).

- Moderation must be accompanied if you consume alcohol products. You should have no more than one daily if you are a woman and only two each day if you are a man.

What Not to Eat

With all the talk of the importance of natural foods, what foods should I avoid to make my intermittent fast more effective?

As a general rule, the following foods should be avoided or at least limited as much as possible.

- *Processed Meats:* While protein is an undeniably important part of a healthy diet, seeking your protein from meats which have been processed will stuff your body so full of chemicals that any benefits the meal might have had are otherwise lost.

  These meats tend to be lower in protein while higher in sodium and preservatives that can cause a variety of health risks, including asthma and heart disease, than the quality of the cuts of meat found in most grocery stores.

- *Non-organic potatoes:* While starch and the carbohydrates they contain are an important part of a balanced meal, non-organic potatoes are not worth the trouble. They are treated with chemicals while still in the ground. They are treated again before they head to the store to ensure they stay "fresh" as long as possible. These chemicals have been shown to increase the risk of health issues like autism, asthma, birth defects, learning disabilities, Parkinson's and Alzheimer's disease as well as multiple types of cancer.

- *Farm-raised salmon:* Much like processed meat, farm-raised salmon are the least healthy type of an otherwise healthy meal choice. When salmon are raised in tubs near one another for a prolonged period of time, they lose much of their natural vitamin D while picking up traces of PCB, DDT, carcinogens, and bromine. Choose wild caught fish if possible.

- *Non-organic milk:* Despite being touted as part of a balanced diet, non-organic milk is routinely found to be full of growth hormones as well as puss as a result of over-milking the cows. The growth hormones leave behind antibiotics which can, in turn, make it more difficult for the human body to counter infections as well as causing an increased chance of colon cancer, prostate cancer, and breast cancer.

- *White Flour:* Much like processed meats, by the time white flour is done being produced; it is completely devoid of any nutritional value. When eaten as part of a regular diet, white flour has been shown to increase a woman's chance of breast cancer by a shocking 200 percent.

These are just a few of the reasons that processed foods should be considered a problem in the modern world. Processed foods can be considered any items which contain preservatives, chemical colors, flavorings, additives or chemicals which change its texture. An additional extremely important warning sign of unhealthy food is when an item contains a large amount of carbohydrates in their refined form.

The cliff-notes version is this, the sooner you begin to take the time to read labels and check ingredients, the sooner you can start getting the most out of the meals you eat in between intermittent fasting sessions. Making a real, consciousness effort to do so may very well be the difference between life and death.

Chapter 6: Intermittent Fasting and Nutrition

How to Boost Your Metabolism

With all the hard work for your intermittent fasting, it is always good to know there are other ways to speed up the process at the same time. It is good to know these are some of the specific foods you should eat to help the metabolism process of losing weight:

Protein-Rich Food Groups

Your body will need more energy to digest these products:

- Eggs

- Seeds and nuts

- Legumes

- Fish

- Meat

- Fish

The thermic effect of food is referred to as TEF which is the number of calories required by your body to absorb/digest the nutrients received by your meals. The protein intake will also make you have a full feeling much longer, and possibly prevent you from overeating.

Essential Vitamins and Minerals

Zinc, iron, and selenium are essential for your healthy body functions. It is shown by research a diet low in these elements reduces the ability of the thyroid gland to produce crucial hormones. This process will significantly slow the metabolism down. It is best to eat seeds, nuts, legumes, meat, and seafood.

- *Chili Peppers:* The chemical found in chili peppers is called capsaicin which will boost your metabolism. The capsaicin will increase the fat and calories you burn during your intermittent fasting plan. Twenty research studies indicated you would lose/burn approximately fifty extra calories daily. However, now all researchers agree with the theory. At any rate, enjoy the chili peppers.

- *Pulses and Legumes:* This food group includes peanuts, lentils, chickpeas, beans, and peas which are extremely high in protein levels in comparison to other plant foods. According to research studies, your higher protein counts will require your body to burn a larger number of calories to digest them, versus the lower-protein foods.

  Recent studies have indicated participants who consumed a legume-rich diet for eight weeks increased the metabolism rate and lost more than 1.5 times more weight versus the other controlled group of applicants.

- *Coffee:* Your caffeine levels can help increase the metabolic rate by approximately 11%. Studies have shown consumption of a minimum of 270 mg of caffeine—about three cups of coffee—will burn away an additional 100 calories daily. The rates can surely boost your intermittent fasting as long as you leave it sugar-free.

- *Tea:* Tea is offered as a good source of beverage because of the catechins in the tea conglomerate with the caffeine to help speed up your metabolism. The catechins are an antioxidant and a type of natural phenol which is from the chemical family of flavonoids. An additional 100 calories can be burned daily to increase your metabolism by four to ten percent with the use of green and oolong tea. The effects may be different with each fasting participant.

Chapter 7: Different Methods for Everyday Living

Method 16:8 or the Leangains Diet Plan

Another term for this plan is the Leangains protocol which implicates for a time slot of eight hours that you can eat a restricted diet and fast for the remainder time of sixteen hours for men and fourteen hours for women. Hugh Jackman was the emblem used to discover the facts and make the headlines.

The 16:8 method for intermittent fasting is the most preferred method for weight loss—besides you will be sleeping for approximately eight of those fasting hours. On the remainder eight to ten hours, the meals should be slightly larger while still relatively health conscious. The fasting period allows for zero calorie consumption.

If you are overweight and have a sedentary lifestyle; you should avoid most of the starchy carbohydrates. You have to cram all of your calories in that time allotment to ensure the successes of the plan. Many individuals on the plan can fit two filling meals into the eight to ten-hour time frame or three regular meals if desired. Once again, the most important element is consistency.

A study was performed by the Obesity Society stating if you have your dinner before 2:00 p.m., your hunger yearnings will be reduced for the remainder of the day. At the same time, your fat-burning reserves are boosted.

No matter what you have heard about this plan, you will not be as hungry once you have the plan and your menu scheduled. That is the secret to a slimmer body, get the counts right. Another advantage is that you can begin the plate at any time that suits your schedule.

You can use these sample menus as a basis for your plan:

Day 1

- **Morning:** Tea, water, or coffee is allowed with a small amount of milk or heavy cream

- **Lunch:** Chicken Breast/black bean sauce, green veggies, and fruit.

- **Dinner:** Salmon and baked veggies with one potato. (If this is too much for one meal, break it in half and eat it later.

Day 2: Repeat Day 1

Additional Tips

- *Sugar Substitutes:* Xylitol can replace sugar. Replace the coffee with black or green tea (advisable if you like the tastes).

- *Stay Hydrated:* Drink plenty of tea, water, or coffee during the morning hours. It also helps prevent the pangs of hunger you will feel. If possible, replace the coffee with black or green tea.

- *Sleep:* You need to have a full eight hours of sleep. It is advisable to avoid your cell phone and laptop (blue light) for up to an hour before you are ready to retire for the evening.

The Consistent Path

The goal is to set your eating schedule to the same time daily to program our body. If you vary during the fasting plan, your hormones will be all over the place, resulting in your body holding onto the weight instead of detaching from the extra pounds.

It is also important to keep your protein on an even kilter throughout your fasting schedule. For women, it should remain at 55 grams daily. For men, it should be in the area of 60 grams daily. If you consume the correct levels of protein and exercise regularly while taking in a steady amount of carbs, you should have all the energy needed on a daily basis.

However, if you are less inclined to exercise you should focus on healthy fats while you minimize the carbs. Aim for approximately 0.7 grams of healthy fats for each pound of body weight daily. As with the other plans, it is best to avoid processed foods and unhealthy fats while searching for healthier—natural alternatives when possible. If you are not an avid exerciser, you also need to adjust your meals for the days to ensure you don't overeat accidentally.

Eat-Stop-Eat

Once or twice each week, you will fast for twenty-four hours. As an illustration, you would eat dinner one morning and not eat again until the following morning. Most professionals say if you make it to twenty hours; it's okay.

To further condition your body, for two days eat about 2,500 calories if you are a man and 2,000 if you are a woman. After several regular eating days, attempt another fasting, and repeat the agenda.

Non-Fasting and Fasting Day Nutrients

For the days on an active fast, try not to consume many calories. You can drink sparkling or plain water, diet soda, coffee, or tea. When the fast is complete, eat what you like using restraint. Enjoy plenty of veggies, fruits, and take advantage of the spices for variety.

Protein should be apparent using twenty to thirty grams of high-quality protein. Consume a total of one-hundred grams every four to five hours. You can use protein powders if needed. If you are gaining extra pounds in between your fasting schedule, consider cutting back by approximately 10% on the amount of food you consume on non-fasting days.

Some individuals cannot 'hack' the plan and state it makes him/her less adaptable to enjoying time with friends at social gatherings. Many have issues of crankiness and headaches which can lead to the plan's failure.

With that said, the plan's benefits are overwhelming because you can judge your progress, and you choose to eat. It takes learning some self-control, but you can get it.

Note: Never fast two consecutive days. Also, you should not take the challenge more than two fasting days in one week.

Fluid Intake

With a strict plan such as this one, you must remain hydrated. You can drink plenty of clear liquids, but where are the nutrients? On your fasting days, stick to apple juice, water, broth, cranberry juice, ice pops, plain gelatin, black coffee or tea. This is okay since you will be fasting for twenty to twenty-four hours.

You can also enjoy foods including ice cream, skim milk, juice with pulp, or strained creamy soup. Try a whey protein supplemental shake or some low-fat frozen yogurt. These choices will provide some essential nutrients, fiber, as well as the necessary calorie counts. Just be sure to use low-calorie juices, ice cream, and a few ice cubes for a smoothie treat.

It is advisable to confer with your physician before you begin this or any other dieting plan. While you are fasting, you might need to discontinue any dietary supplements or medications. According to research at Vanderbilt University, daily liquid diets will provide you between 400 to 800 calories.

Additional Tips

With this fasting method, it is essential to not fall into a habit of fasting and binging because it will create havoc within your body. It is more than your body can handle since the cycle will only work for individuals who can practice control and moderate consumption of food. It is recommended by the professionals to perform resistance-style weight training on the days you aren't fasting.

Try a minimal yoga session or light cardio exercise if you feel completely out of it on your fasting days. Any more vigorous exercising could make it difficult to achieve the time allotment of your fasting schedule. Remember, at first—it is common to feel angered, anxious, fatigued, or have headaches. This will pass once your body adjusts to the new dieting plan.

Try to keep in mind that every single day you can successfully stay on your desired plan is one more day toward your successful goal.

The Warrior Diet

It is believed that the name of the diet is a reflection of the ancient ancestors who were natural nocturnal eaters. As a step up from the Leangains diet and as a variation of the daily fast; the Warrior Diet is a plan promoting one healthy meal daily—usually dinner. The method is parallel with the human 24-hour rhythm and can encourage excellent general health while removing the harmful toxins from your body. You should try to eat at least several hours before going to sleep for the night.

The Daytime Feeding Schedule

For the plan to be effective, you need to consume less food during the daytime hours. Eat small servings of veggies, fruits, and a protein such as a yogurt, whey protein, or kefir. Sidestep consumption of meats, grains, refined foods (pasta, corn tortillas, etc.) which lack the nutrient and are usually processed foods. Also, avoid sugary beverages and treats.

Every few hours, you should eat a small serving of protein or fruit. Eat green veggies such as celery, leafy greens, cucumbers, and peppers which are not restricted to your intake amounts.

Nighttime Feeding Frenzy

You can eat as much food as you wish but keep the correct food combinations. Enlist as many different aromas, colors, and textures to create new taste sensations for your evening meal. Eliminate or avoid using white vinegar. When you feel full or have satisfied your hunger or if you become more thirsty than hungry; it is time to stop eating.

Follow the Rules

Start off with your salad, protein, and veggies and complete the meal with a few fats or carbs. Take a short twenty-minute break after the protein and vegetables which will be a signal to your brain to recharge your appetite. If you are still hungry, continue your meal.

Organic foods are the best choices which will include grass-fed, free range, and hormone free animal products. Your eggs, dairy, and meat, as well as your fish consumption, should be a 'wild' catch.

Processed sugars are considered toxic on this diet plan.

You should also exercise as a critical step in your fasting plan. After your workout, consume 20 to 30 grams of net protein with no additional sugar.

Guidelines for Success

Remember to plan your menus ahead of time to be sure you have the right combination of foods. Vegetables and protein will combine with your entire menu planning needs. Starch, sugar, and fat cannot conglomerate effectively.

Examples of the Right Combinations

- Eggs and beans
- Seeds and nuts
- Eggs and potatoes
- Berries and Whey protein
- Cocoa nibs and peanut butter
- Potatoes and peas
- Nuts and wine

- Cheese and wine
- Rice and beans

Examples of the Wrong Combinations

- Pasta and wine
- Pasta and nuts
- Raisins and nuts (trail mix)
- Sugar and cream
- Jelly and peanut butter
- Jam and bread
- Granola (honey nut)
- Sour cream and potatoes

Sample Plan: Daytime Options

Early Morning: Tea, coffee, or cacao (no sugar) whole milk

Mid-morning: Vegetable juice or one fruit (8 ounces of berries)

Lunchtime: Salad with tomatoes, peppers, mixed greens, mushroom, onions, sprouts, and cucumber

Dressing for the salad: Use a small amount of olive oil OR whey protein

Afternoon: Fresh Fruit or Vegetable juice

Sample Plan: Nighttime Meal

For your one large meal of the day try some of the following food groups:

Protein: Eggs (cooked or poached), wild catch fish, organic cheeses such as goat and cottage

*Cooked Veggies***:** Grilled or steamed cauliflower, broccoli, zucchini, onion, spinach, okra, and mushroom

Raw Veggies: Broccoli sprouts, salad greens, as well as red, yellow, and orange vegetables

Carbs: Use puree from butternut squash, carrots, Brussels sprouts, turnips, pumpkin, or cauliflower (steamed rooted veggies)

Use modest amounts of aged cheese, olive paste, parmesan cheese, or goat feta to top off your protein and vegetables. During the detox meals, you can also reduce stress with green tea and berberine. The berberine is a supplement to help unlock your metabolism to help balance your blood sugar levels during the detox diet plan.

The warrior diet is one of the most popular plans because it allows a sensible number of snacks to the daily routine which makes it more appealing to beginners on the fasting path. The amount of energy will naturally get your body in the habit of burning fat for fuel.

Every-Other-Day Diet Plan

The alternate days using this plan was established by an assistant professor, Dr. Krista Varady, from the University of Illinois. Women should consume between 500 to 600 calories, and men need to consume more than 400 to 500 calories daily. However, on the feast day, you can eat anything you want and as much as you want.

The plan takes some planning since the diet begins between the hours of noon and 2 pm. These are some of the items to make your day more enjoyable:

The following meal will supply you with roughly 475 calories—depending on the type of soup used.

- ½ cup cooked chicken cooked without the skin and topped/Lemon juice/Fresh-ground pepper

- Bowl of tomato or low-sodium vegetable soup

- 1 ¼ cups of fruit salad

For Men Only: You can have a whole-wheat roll (medium 96-calorie) for a total of 566 calories.

Prepare the salad with pears strawberries, mandarin orange segments, and melon.

Enjoy Lean Beef
Choose a lean piece of beef cut similar to sirloin or tenderloin steak, and enjoy some low-calorie side dishes. The basics of the plan are calculated for women. For men, add 80 additional calories with a one-cup serving of asparagus with a teaspoon of olive oil for the topping.

For the remainder of the meal, enjoy a three-ounce seared steak with some onions. Top it off with a bit of blue cheese. Serve it with one cup of chard sautéed in 1 teaspoon of olive oil along with a ½ cup of polenta (cornmeal). Use some lemon juice for seasoning.

Substitute with Seafood:
You need to consume some omega-3 fatty acids to remain heart-healthy. For men, boost the counts to 553 by enjoying one cup of kale that has been sautéed with olive oil for an additional 102 calories. Flavor the kale with crushed red pepper, red wine vinegar, and garlic.

For a woman (451 calories) enjoy three ounces of sautéed shrimp with jalapenos, garlic, onions, and some tomatoes (fresh and diced) on a bed of ½ cup of brown rice. Place it all in a six-inch corn tortilla. Also, have ¼ of an avocado (chopped) for dessert.

The Choice of No Meat:
Women can choose a meatless meal with 473 calories using a whole-wheat pizza crust. As toppings use some black beans, diced tomatoes, barbecue sauce, fresh corn, and shredded mozzarella cheese. Have a bowl of butternut squash soup, made using ¾ cup of fruit sorbet and veggie stock.

Men can veg-out with one cup of cauliflower salad for an extra 48 calories using reduced-fat mayonnaise. He could also add ½ cup fruit such as blueberries, ½ cup yogurt if desired. It is best to use the lower fat plain yogurt with the meal.

A Week's Worth of Planning

The logic behind this weekly regimen example involves eating 300 calories on the low-calorie days but can increase to 400 calories if you have an exercise plan in motion. On the brighter side; women can eat 1200 to 1800 calories on the usual days.

The Low-Calorie Count Days

Day One:

Breakfast

- 1 small slice of deli meat
- 1 six-ounce glass of tomato juice
- ½ cup strawberries

Morning Snack Time
- ¼ cup mixed berries
- 1 tablespoon whey protein
- Blend the ingredients with 3 ice cubes and a cup of water

Lunch
- 1-ounce low-fat cheese
- ½ cup of pickles
- 1-six-ounce cup of tomato juice

Afternoon Snack Time
- 1 tablespoon salad dressing (calorie-free) on one celery stalk
-

Dinner Time
- Make an omelet using three egg whites, mushrooms, green peppers, and onions.
- For dessert have ½ cup of strawberries

Evening Snack
- Whey protein smoothie is your savior to enjoy with a cup of mixed veggies.

Normal Calorie Counted Days

Day 2:

Breakfast
- 1 small banana
- 20 Blueberries
- 1 English muffin (whole wheat) with 2 ¼ teaspoons of peanut butter
- 2/3 cup fat-free yogurt

Morning Snack Time
- 3 saltines
- 1 reduced-fat string cheese stick

Lunch
- 3 tablespoons of hummus with tomato and lettuce
- 1 Whole wheat wrap
- *Dessert*: 1 cup low-fat yogurt and ½ cup of applesauce

Afternoon Snack Time
- 15 almonds

Dinner
- 3 ounces—chicken breast
- 1 cup of broccoli and 2/3 cup of couscous

Evening Snacks
- 1 tablespoon peanut butter on 2 large graham cracker squares

Low-Calorie Day

Day 3:

Breakfast Meal
- ½ fruit serving
- 1-ounce of protein
- 1 six-ounce glass of tomato juice

Mid-morning Snack
- ¼ of a serving of fruit
- *Smoothie:* Combine three pieces of ice + one cup of water with one tablespoon whey protein.

Lunch Menu
- 1-ounce of protein
- 1 six-ounce glass of tomato juice

Mid-afternoon Snack
- Enjoy something under 50 calories.

Dinner Meal
- No more than 100 calories—include protein, veggies, and fruit as a focus point

Normal Calorie Count Day

Day 4:

Breakfast Meal
- 20 blueberries
- ¼ cup banana
- Whole wheat English muffin with 1 tablespoon of peanut butter

Mid-morning Snack
- 2 tablespoons of light cheese
- 3 rye crackers

Lunch
- 6 whole wheat crackers
- 1 cup of vegetable beef soup
- 1 piece fresh fruit

Mid-Afternoon Snack
- 5-6 medium strawberries
- 1-ounce dark chocolate

Dinner Menu
Steak and Peppers

Grill or broil:
1—four-ounce flank steak flavored with pepper and salt

Sauté Pepper Mixture:
2 teaspoons red wine
1 teaspoon olive oil
¼ cup onion sliced
¾ cup sliced bell pepper
1 tablespoon hoisin sauce

Instructions
1. Over a medium heat setting, sauté each of the ingredients listed using the teaspoon of olive oil.
2. After the flank steak is cooked to your preference, add the sautéed pepper mixture.

Calories: 267 per serving

Method 5:2 and 4:3

For this plan, you would eat a regular diet for five days. For the remaining two days, you will eat approximately 500 to 600 calories. The baseline of the calorie ingestion is 2,000 for women and 2,500 for men. A few famous names swear by the diet including Jennifer Aniston and David Cameron. These are some of the ways of how to manage the 5:2 diet plan. Just remember carbs don't mix with your fasting days.

Experiment with Mealtime

- Test different eating times. It doesn't always have to be an early time of day when you aren't hungry. You can wait a bit longer if you wish.

- Change from eating three meals each day to two such as having brunch. It can combine the meals and save the calories. Try having brunch around 11 am and dinner at 7 pm, or even a larger meal at 8 pm with your significant other.

Maximize the Flavoring and Minimize the Calories

- Soups are a respectable choice—also proven by research—because you remain full longer than just a modest serving of veggies on a plate.

- Flavor your foods with spices and herbs such as these—lemon juice or vinegar for salads or curry pastes or chili flakes in stews, baked beans, or soups.

- Go for the veggies and salads with smaller servings of fish, eggs, lean meat, or tofu.

Use Fresh Ingredients

- Not only are you eating better and healthier products, but also most fresh ingredients are less expensive. Search for seasonal produce for the most savings.

- Search for items such as a tomato that have ripened. These will make a yummy treat with a few of your special herbs and balsamic vinegar. You could also add it to some soup.

- During the winter months, experiment with butternut squash or parsnip—roasted—with low-fat feta—or in soup.

- Cut some peppers in half and stuff them with cream cheese, tuna, or similar ingredients and grill them. You can add an egg to the mix for a taste challenge.

Food for the Fasting Days

- Berries and natural yogurt

- Plentiful veggie portions

- Baked or boiled eggs

- Low-calorie cup soups

- Other soups: vegetable, tomato, miso, cauliflower

- Lean mean or grilled fish

- Tea or black coffee

- Water (sparkling or still)

The 4:3 Diet Plan

Health benefits include asthma relief, reduction in heart arrhythmias, insulin resistance, menopausal hot flashes, seasonal allergies, and much more. After twelve weeks of fasting using the 4:3 method diet plan, these are the results from a small study group:

- Fat mass reduction: 3.5 kg with no muscle mass

  changes

- Body weight reduction: Over 5 kg

- Increased LDL particle size

- Reduced blood levels: 20% reduction of triglycerides

- Leptin levels: 40% decreased

- Levels CRP: Reduced levels (inflammation marker in

  your body)

How the 4:3 Diet Plan is Different from the 5:2 Plan

The 5:2 intermittent fasting choices are much simpler than the 4:3 Plan because you are more restricted. You will be intermittently fasting for three out of the seven days. You should not eat processed/sugary/refined foods for four of the days. If you do, your body will crave the supplementary fatty acids you need to thrive.

If you consume junk on those four days, you will defeat the purpose of the plan. Just remember, not to over-indulge. As you train your body by eating a well-planned diet; your body will adjust to the routine, and you won't feel as hungry.

The 4:3 Plan acclaims you skip the morning meal, and it recommends you check your weight daily. However, this can be disheartening if your weight fluctuates.

A sample plan for the 4:3 method of weight loss is as follows:

- *Breakfast:* Eat nothing.

- *Lunch:* Leek, lentil, or chicken soup with a snack such as a small tangerine

- *Dinner:* A side salad using lemon juice as the dressing with some salt, pepper, or similar seasonings along with a small lean fillet of grilled chicken

- *Snacks:* Veggies or fruit

You can have a light breakfast if you enjoy a morning meal, but you will need to eliminate the snack during the day. You can also skip lunch, and have a larger breakfast. This is more challenging to follow than the 5:2 intermittent fasting plan because you have three days you can only consume 500 calories versus two days on the 5:2 diet.

Suggestions for the Fasting Days Using the 4:3 Method

- Drink an abundance of water.

- Drink coffee and tea for an additional boost.

- Consume a 400-calorie meal with a snack of 100 total calories.

- Chew sugar-free gum to fight the hunger spurts.

If you have a busy lifestyle, you can cheat once in a while with a low-calorie pre-packaged meal. (This is not a regular outlet.)

The point in both plans is to eat as much as you want and not feel deprived on the days you can eat normally—just do it in moderation, not over-indulgence.

Chapter 8: Tips and Simple Meal Plans

Simple Guidelines to Follow for Fasting

Stay in Control: Depending on which method you choose for your intermittent fasting routine, you need to ask the question if you can follow the crucial diet plans involved to keep your food intake at proper levels. If you are attempting to achieve a 500-calorie debit daily, you have to keep your appetite under control, because a single missed meal won't provide a generous window for the next meal.

Keep a Calorie Tally Record: You must keep an accurate record of your calorie intake because if you are not careful, you can easily overeat at mealtime. If your goal is to work off more calories than you consume to lose the one pound of weight you want to lose each week.

Stay with the Chosen Plan: You need to get into the habit of setting a regular schedule for your fasting plan. Once your body adjusts to the specific method, it will become confused if you try another plan. For example, if you are on the 5:2 plan and switch to the 16:8 plan, your body will stop the weight loss until it can readjust to the new plan. You will lose valuable time by switching. Consistency is essential for a successful fasting plan.

Breakfasts and Snacks

While you are attempting to lose weight on the intermittent fasting plan, you should not feel the need to be hungry no matter which of the procedures you decide to use. Some of the recipes call for grams which need to be converted to ounces. Use this handy chart to calculate the amounts.

This chapter is dedicated to some of the meals you can use. Each menu plan has a calorie count within the recipe.

Breakfast

Porridge

89 Calories: 25 g Porridge oats
10 Calories: ½ teaspoon honey
0 Calories: Water and Cinnamon

Tips:
Instead of milk, use some water to reduce the calorie count. For some additional flavor add just a pinch of cinnamon. You can also improve the meal with a few nuts if you add the calories to your plan.

Toast and Beans

55 Calories: 1 slice whole- meal bread (small loaf size)
42 Calories: 50 g Baked beans

For a quick and low-calorie choice, tempt your taste buds with this unique idea.

Fruity Breakfast Meals

Watermelon

The natural sugars are more beneficial than a cereal bar.
96 Calories: 300 g serving

Honey and Bananas

10 Calories: ½ teaspoon honey
89 Calories: 1 small banana

Apricots and Yogurt

68 Calories: Two chopped apricots and 25 g Greek yogurt (low-fat)

Apricots, Greek Fat-Free Yogurt, and Mixed Berries

24 Calories: 3 tablespoons Greek yogurt
17 Calories: 1 Apricot
19 Calories: 50 g Raspberries
16 Calories: 50 g Strawberries
20 Calories: 50 g Blackberries
Total Calories: 96

Blend the ingredients for a yummy treat.

Greek Yogurt, Sultanas, & Almonds

24 Calories: 3 tablespoons Greek Yogurt (fat-free)
42 Calories: 1 tablespoon sultanas
28 Calories: 4 almonds (whole)
Total Calorie Intake: 94

Blueberries, Kiwi, & Greek Yogurt

42 Calories: 1 kiwi (chopped)
29 Calories: Blueberries (50g)
24 Calories: 3 tablespoons yogurt
Total Intake: 95 Calories

Mix all the ingredients for a tasty meal.

Raspberry and Cranberry Smoothie

14 ounces/175 g raspberries
7 ounces cranberry juice
 3 ounces natural yogurt
Mint sprigs

For a quick and easy breakfast try this one packing 100 calories per serving.
Serves 4 to 6 people

Eggs for Breakfast

Plain Eggs

100 Calories: 1 large boiled egg
Add a slice of wheat toast with two small poached eggs for a 188-calorie delight.

Scrambled with Mushrooms

78 Calories: 1 medium egg
13 Calories: fresh chopped mushrooms (100 g)
Total Count: 91 Calories

Scramble the ingredients and enjoy!

Spinach Omelet

16 Calories: 60 g fresh spinach
78 Calories: 1 medium egg
Total Calorie Count: 94

Instructions
1. Simply, beat/whisk the egg and place in a frying pay.
2. When the bottom is cooked; add spinach to the top and grill.
3. If you want, you can add some herbs, salt, or pepper for additional flavoring.

Ham Omelet

19 Calories: 1 slice of ham/wafer sliced
78 Calories: 1 Egg (medium)

Prepare the ingredients as above.

Starchy Options

Bread with Honey

55 Calories: 1 slice bread (whole meal from a small loaf)

40 Calories: 2 teaspoons honey
Total: 95

Perfect Pancakes

2 eggs
1 1/3 cups milk (300 ml) 100 g all-purpose flour
Sunflower Oil

Instructions
Blend the ingredients, cook, and sprinkle with a splash of lemon juice.

114 Calories: Per serving
Total Servings: 4

Pancake Variation

2 whole eggs
1 ripe banana

Instructions
1. Simply blend the two ingredients until the bananas are completely mashed.
2. Gently grease a pan with a sprinkle of oil and add the batter.
3. Cook 20 to 30 seconds, flip them over and enjoy.

Calorie counts: 1 medium banana/118 g/105 calories
                    2 large eggs/100 g/156 calories

A total of 261 calories is not bad for these yummy delights!

In Advance: Fiber-Packed Cereal

If you have a busy lifestyle and always rush in the morning, consider making this tasty breakfast bowl. It will serve 18 meals at 124 calories each.

100 g All-bran
300 g jumbo oats

50 g golden linseed
25 g wheat germ
140 g ready-to-eat apricots (chunked)
100 g dark raisins

Instructions
1. Blend all the ingredients.
2. Ahead of time break down each of the units and store in airtight containers.
3. To serve: Add milk and let it soak. Grate some unpeeled apple over it for a flavor delight.

Note: The cereal can be safely stored for two months in the airtight container.

Snacks

Snack time doesn't always have to be boring. You can trick your mind by using the small plate. Add some of these healthier choices to your intermittent fasting meal plan for weight loss. You will also notice the 'not so healthy' choices are higher calorie content, but that is the advantage of planning your menu before you are hungry. Each of these yummy delights will keep you going until lunchtime.

130 Calories: One square dark chocolate and a small banana

55 Calories: 10 g of 85% Dark chocolate

75 Calories: 3 Stuffed celery sticks with low-fat cottage cheese

96 Calories: 16 olives (green or black)

90 Calories: 1 Cup Cherries

29 Calories: 100 g Honeydew melon

42 Calories: 2 Satsumas/tangerine (The Christmas Orange)

90 Calories: 3 thin slices Pineapple

61 Calories: 100 g Grapes/ OR 100 Calories: 30 grapes

42 Calories: Sun-Maid Mini Box of Raisins

90 Calories: 25 Pistachio nuts

74 Calories: 10 Salted peanuts

Each Item Counts as 100 Calories:

31 Asparagus Spears

9—5" Spears of Broccoli

16 ribs Celery

12 Raw Brussels Sprouts

28 Baby Carrots

82 Red Kidney Beans

60 Raw Green Beans

43 Boiled or Steamed Okra Pods

100 Radishes

20 Sun-Dried Tomatoes

22 Cloves Garlic

100 Raspberries

5 Dried Figs

6 Dried Apricots

8 Cashew Nuts

10 Pringles Chips

21 Pretzels Unsalted Minis

4 Sardines in Oil Drained

13 Large Boiled or Steamed Shrimp

15 pieces Dry-Roasted Cashew Halves

Tasty Beverages Too Good to Pass Up!

Starbucks Grande Skinny Iced Latte: 96 Calories

Avocado—Chocolate Milkshake: 169 Total Calories/2 servings

Simply blend and enjoy:
1 ½ cups skim milk
2 tablespoons each:
  - Brown sugar
  - Cocoa powder
½ ripe avocado
1 teaspoon vanilla extract

These are just a few of the tasty treats you can have in store for you while you are on the intermittent fasting diet plan. There are many more for you to discover that will have you losing weight and toning those muscles to get fit in no time!

Conclusion

Thank you again for downloading *Intermittent Fasting: Lose Fat, Build Muscle and Get Fit*! I hope it provided you with the understanding of the wide variety of options you have when it comes to intermittent fasting and how you can best mix and match to find the perfect solution for you. Making the decision to alter your primary eating patterns is a major one, and it is important that you take the full weight of the decision into account before acting.

If you are convinced that you have what it takes to take full advantage of the benefits that intermittent fasting has to offer, then the next step is to stop reading, and to start fasting. Choose the type of intermittent fasting that seems like the best fit for you and give it a try.

Try not to become discouraged if you don't receive immediate results. Make an effort to find the one that's right for you. Above all, don't rush, and remember, intermittent fasting is a marathon not a sprint, slow and steady will win the race.

Lastly, if you found this book useful in any way, a review on Amazon is always appreciated!

Description

Do you always find yourself on the lookout for new diets, but lose interest when they prove to be too much of a hassle, and more trouble than they're worth? If this sounds like you, then *Intermittent Fasting: Lose Fat, Build Muscle and Get Fit* is the book you have been waiting for. Inside, you will find everything you need to look and feel better than you have in years.

Intermittent fasting is a new lifestyle designed to ensure that you get the most out of every meal you eat. The idea is that you don't need to change what you are eating. You just need to change how often you are eating it. Simply by working with your body's natural rhythms, you can start seeing real gains in terms of weight loss and muscle built in as little as one month.

Inside you will find:

1. Everything you need to know to start intermittent fasting immediately and getting the most out of it in the process.

2. Several types of intermittent fasting means there is bound to be one that's right for you.

3. Many ways are shown to ensure you start intermittently fasting properly and stick with it long term.

What are you waiting for? Why not get started on the path to a healthier you today!

www.ingramcontent.com/pod-product-compliance
Lightning Source LLC
Chambersburg PA
CBHW071130280526
45787CB00003B/1231